Essential Oils For Beginners: Essential Oil Recipes For Beginners

How to Use Essential Oils To Heal Your Body And Treat Your Hair, Skin And Mind

Table of Contents

Introduction

I want to thank you and congratulate you for purchasing the book, *"Essential Oils For Beginners: Essential Oil Recipes For Beginners - How to Use Essential Oils To Heal Your Body And Treat Your Hair, Skin And Mind"*

The use of essential oils is gaining in popularity and for good reason. Essential oils have antibacterial, antifungal, and antioxidant properties making them very useful for a healthy body. Have you heard a lot about essential oils but don't know where to start? Do you know the amazing health problems that essential oils can address but don't know where to start? Are you looking for a comprehensive guide with as many essential oil recipes as possible to help you address various problems? If this is what you are looking for, then this is the book for you. This book has over 60 essential oil recipes for healthy hair and skin and to treat your body and mind. This book will help you learn of various ways of using essential oils to enjoy their amazing healing properties.

Thanks again and I hope you enjoy this book!

Essential Oils 101

Essential oils occur naturally and are liquids extracted from stems, leaves, flowers, barks, roots and other plant components. They are highly concentrated and contain the true essence of the plants source, possessing strong medicinal and cosmetic qualities. Most essential oils are high in antibacterial, antifungal, and antiviral properties and they do not accumulate in the body over time but are excreted after performing their function. When using essential oils, especially when applying them topically on their skin, you need to dilute them with carrier oils, waxes, alcohols, butters, since they are usually very concentrated.

Carrier oils are vegetable oils derived from the fatty portion of a plant and mostly from nuts, seeds, and kernels. These include oils extracted from almonds, borage, camellia, hemp, sesame, sunflower, pomegranate, watermelon, grape and cranberry seeds, apricot kernel, fractionated coconut, macadamia nut, hazel nut, kukui nut, and peanut, olive oil, jojoba, evening primrose, and pecan rose hip oils.

As earlier indicated, essential oils can be applied topically on the skin whose semi-permeability allows absorption of the active chemicals in essential oils. Different factors affect the absorption of essential oils through the skin. For instance, applying heat and massages increase circulation and absorption of essential oils on the affected area. Additionally, absorption is high in certain skin areas containing numerous sweat glands and hair follicles, such as the head, genitals, palms, soles and armpits.

I cannot emphasize how important it is to dilute essential oils before use. This is because since they are very concentrated, undiluted essential oils will result in adverse skin reactions. However, a few essential oils are generally recognized as safe to use undiluted. These essential oils include German chamomile, tea tree, lavender, rose geranium and sandalwood. However, remember to use these oils sparingly.

It is important to note however that undiluted essential oils should never be used on a child because of their more delicate skin, which tends to be very sensitive to the potency of essential oils. Only use half of the essential oil recommended in the recipe when used on children. Essential oils safe for babies include; Cypress, Frankincense, Geranium, Ginger, Rosemary, Rosewood, Sandalwood and Lavender. Here is a list of 19 essential oils that are safe for babies and children.

Use essential oils cautiously during pregnancy and when nursing. Avoid essential oils like Wormseed, Wintergreen, Thuja, Pennyroyal, rosemary, ginger, Myrrh, Jasmine, Hyssop, and Boldo leaf. Read more on pregnancy and essential oils.

It is always important to test the essential oil by performing a skin patch test before applying it. You can test if you're sensitive to an essential oil before using it by combining one drop of essential oil with ½ teaspoon carrier oil then rub this on the inside, upper portion of your arm and wait a few hours and if no redness or itching develops, you're most likely not sensitive to that essential oil. Stay away from any oil extract of a plant you are allergic to.

How To Use Essential Oils

Essential oils can be inhaled through the nose or mouth. Inhaled essential oils affect the brain resulting into profound physiological and psychological effects. Often, essential oils are put in a diffuser for inhalation. Common examples include inhaling some eucalyptus essential oil whenever you have a cough or inhaling peppermint essential oil when you want to deal with reduce nausea or fatigue, smelling rosemary essential oil to help memory recall and performance on tests. Additionally, inhaling ylang-ylang, peppermint, lavender, chamomile, grapefruit and lemon, help promote a good mood. You can also ingest essential oils. Oral ingestion of essential oils is only recommended when specially trained physicians and pharmacists recommend and administer them because intense knowledge and expertise is required for safe practice. Applying essential oils topically is also a great way of making use of an essential oil to enjoy its benefits. Always remember that you need to make use of an essential oil that is pure.

In order to test purity of the essential oil, put a single drop of it on a piece of construction paper. If it evaporates very quickly without leaving any noticeable ring this means that it is pure. If there is a ring left, it is most likely diluted by the manufacturer with oil.

Most essential oils will last for at least 5-10 years. However, citrus oils reduce in potency after a year or two. Store your essential oils in dark glass bottles and out of direct sunlight to preserve their potency.

Several essential oils should be avoided even through skin contact for example bitter almond, Calamus, Camphor and Pennyroyal. You can read more on **toxic essential oils.**

Essential Oils To Treat Your Skin

Essential Oil Recipes For Treatment Of Acne

Essential oils provide a great alternative to the use of harsh chemicals that prescription medication and acne creams contain. Essential oils can protect your skin from bacteria that causes acne, alleviate mild to moderate acne, reduce excess oiliness, and speed up the healing process during and after an outbreak.

Here are some recipes that can help in treating acne. Refer to this blend every time it's mentioned in a recipe.

Acne Treatment Blend

Ingredients

20 drops of lavender essential oil

30 drops of lemon essential oil

30 drops of tea tree essential oil

Instructions

Mix all ingredients in a dark bottle then shake well before use.

Poppy Face Scrub

Ingredients

20 drops of 'essential oil acne treatment blend'

250ml poppy seeds (or finely grounded oatmeal)

125ml vegetable oils (jojoba and almond oil)

Instructions

Mix all the ingredients in a wide jar and cover with a tight lid then massage the mixture on your face lightly avoiding the sensitive eye region then rinse with tepid water. Don't scrub your face if you have acne wounds.

Castile Facial Cleanser

Ingredients

50 drops of the 'acne treatment blend '

2 ounces jojoba oil

2 ounces of natural aloe Vera gel

8 ounces liquid castile soap

Instructions

Mix all the ingredients in a pump bottle and use is as a facial cleanser once daily.

Flour Face Scrub

Ingredients

250ml almond flour, grain flour or gram flour

125ml vegetable oils (like jojoba or sweet almond oil)

20 drops of the "essential oil acne treatment blend"

Instructions

Mix all the ingredients in a tightly covered jar. Apply mixture on face avoiding sensitive eye regions then rinse with tepid water.

Fruity Face Mask

Ingredients

1 teaspoon pineapple, papaya puree, fresh lemon juice or water

3 drops of the "essential oil acne treatment blend"

2 teaspoons of cosmetic clay like French green clay, multanimitti clay, rhassoul clay or glacial clay.

Instructions

Mix all ingredients to make a smooth paste then apply on your face avoiding eye region. Allow it dry for some time then rinse with tepid water.

Milk Face Scrub

Ingredients

20 drops of "essential oil acne treatment blend"

125 ml vegetable oils (like sweet almonds and jojoba oil)

250ml milk powder or yogurt powder

Instructions

Mix all the ingredients in a tightly covered jar. Apply mixture on face avoiding sensitive eye regions then rinse with warm water. Avoid scrubbing on lesions.

Honey Face Facial Cleanser

Ingredients

2 teaspoons of yogurt

3 teaspoons of honey

5 drops of 'acne treatment blend'

Instructions

Mix all the ingredients and massage on the blemishes then rinse with warm water after some time.

Facial Toner

Ingredients

20 drops "essential oil acne treatment blend"

100ml distilled water

Instructions

Add the blend to water. Use the mixture as your facial toner.

Herbal Face Scrub

Ingredients

20 drops of 'essential oil acne treatment blend'

1 tablespoon dry, ground herbs (witch hazel, rose flower petals or lavender flowers)

1 teaspoon spices (like turmeric powder, cinnamon powder)

250 ml finely ground oatmeal

125ml vegetable oils (like sweet almond, jojoba oils)

Instructions

Mix all in a wide tightly covered jar. Massage the mixture on face avoiding the eyes then rinse with tepid water after some time. Avoid scrubbing areas with lesions.

Anti-Aging Serum

Ingredients

1 teaspoon vitamin e oil

3 drops of carrot seed essential oil

3 drops "essential oil acne treatment blend"

1 ounce jojoba oil

Instructions

Mix all the ingredients in a dark bottle with a dropper top. Mix the ingredients properly by rolling on your palm. Apply on affected areas. This blend is helpful in treating acne and getting rid of acne scars.

Clay Face Scrub

Ingredients

125ml vegetable oils (like jojoba or sweet almond oil)

20 drops of the "essential oil acne treatment blend"

250ml bentonite clay or rhassoul clay or multanimitti

Instructions

Mix all the ingredients in a tightly covered jar. Apply mixture on face avoiding sensitive eye regions then rinse with tepid water.

Herbal Face Mask

Ingredients

1 teaspoon of water or natural aloe Vera gel

3 drops of essential oil "essential oil acne treatment blend"

1 teaspoon powdered spices or herbs (like rose flower petals, witch hazel, turmeric powder or lavender flowers, lemongrass and cinnamon powder)

Instructions

Mix all ingredients to make a smooth paste then apply on your face avoiding eye region. Let it sit for 15 minutes then rinse with tepid water.

Facial Steamer

Ingredients

50 drops "essential oil acne treatment blend"

250 ml water

Instructions

Add the two ingredients and use the mixture in a facial steamer.

Facial Massage Oil

20 drops "essential oil acne treatment blend"

125ml jojoba oil

Instructions

Add the blend to jojoba oil and create massage oil with healing properties.

Acne Treatment Blend

Ingredients

7 drops tea tree

30 ml jojoba oil

10 drops lavender

3 drops geranium

Instructions

Put jojoba in a dark glass bottle and add the rest of the essential oils. Close the bottle tightly then shake to mix oils. Apply a small amount on the affected area twice daily. Avoid the eyes, nose and lips and gently shake before use. Be patient as you wait for results. If you don't like the smell of tea tree, substitute with lemon grass. You can also use aloe Vera gel in place of jojoba oil.

Natural Exfoliating Scrub With Essential Oil

Ingredients

2 - 3 teaspoons raw oats (not the pre-cooked type)

¼ teaspoon of apple cider vinegar

1 drop of basil oil

Pure honey as needed

Instructions

Crush the dry oats into smaller bits either by hand or in a grinder. Mix the dry oats with pure honey and ¼ teaspoon of apple cider vinegar until it forms a smooth mixture. Add more honey as required. Then add 1 drop of basil oil to the mixture.

You can replace the basil oil with tea tree oil for a skin problem to promote the healing process.

After washing and drying the face with a towel, you can now apply it using gentle circular movements while ensuring that you avoid the eye area. Leave this mixture on for about 15 minutes and wash off with lots of tepid water. Produces excellent results and is affordable.

Essential Oil Recipes For Treating Psoriasis

Essential oils are effective in healing and preventing psoriasis lesions owing to their detoxifying and antibacterial properties. Here are great recipes that will help in treating psoriasis.

Alkalyzing Hydrotherapy Bath

Ingredients

1 cup oats

1 cup baking soda

1 cup corn flour

Warm water

1 cup apple cider vinegar

Instructions

Put the oats, baking soda and corn flour in a pop sock and tie properly. Put the loaded pop sock in warm water and add apple cider vinegar. Squeeze the sock well. Use this bath 5 times a week to help smooth and heal your body.

Moisturizing Bath

Ingredients

4 drops lavender

1 teaspoon of virgin cold pressed olive oil

4 drops bergamot

½ cup Dead Sea salt

1 cup oats

2 drops German chamomile

1 teaspoon jojoba oil

Instructions

Put all the ingredients in pop sock and tie properly. Add the soak to warm water and squeeze regularly to ensure the salts dissolve and oat milk is released. Use this bath blend once or twice a week to help moisturize and soothe skin and help prevent infections.

Magnesium Bath

Ingredients

1 cup of Himalayan salt

1-3 cups of magnesium flakes and Epsom salts

10-25 drops lavender or mint essential oil

1 teaspoon vanilla extract

Instructions

Mix all ingredients and add to warm bath water. Use daily.

Moisturizing Aloe Vera Gel/Cream

Ingredients

100 ml of moisturizing cream base or seaweed and aloe Vera gel

10 ml bergamot

10ml vitamin E oil

10ml avocado oil

3 drops German chamomile

4 ml tea tree

10ml jojoba oil

4 ml patchouli

10 ml lavender

Instructions

Stir well and keep in an airtight jar. Use after a shower or bath. Apply on lesions or places the lesions are likely to appear.

Famous Essential Oil Recipe For Psoriasis

Ingredients

9 drops bergamot oil

6 tablespoons carrier oil (like avocado oil, sweet almond oil or pumpkin seed oil)

1 drop ylang ylang oil

11 drops lavender oil

3 drops mandarin oil

1 drop clary sage oil

10 drops frankincense oil

10 drops geranium oil

4 drops patchouli oil

Instructions

Add the carrier oil of choice into a glass bottle with a dropper. Add the essential oils then put the lid on. Gently shake the bottle to mix the ingredients. Use this blend on your lesions twice daily.

Essential Oil Recipes For Treating Eczema

These great essential oil recipes will help in the healing and prevention of eczema.

Homemade Eczema Cream

Ingredients

¼ cup shea butter

¼ cup coconut oil (soft or melted)

25 drops of Melrose essential oil

15 drops of lavender essential oil

½ teaspoon vitamin E oil

Instructions

In a small bowl mix coconut oil, vitamin E oil, shea butter and whisk well. Add the essential oils and stir until combined. Transfer to a container and store at room temperature. Apply on the affected area daily or when the rash appears.

Magnesium Bath

Ingredients

½ cup of Himalayan salt

1-2 cup of magnesium flakes and Epsom salts

10-15 drops lavender or mint essential oil

½ teaspoon vanilla extract

Instructions

Mix all ingredients and add to warm bath water. Use daily.

Homemade Herbal Slave

Ingredients

2 tablespoons dried comfrey leaf

2 tablespoons dried plantain leaf (herb not banana)

1 teaspoon dried Echinacea root (optional)

1 tablespoon dried calendula flowers (optional)

2 cups olive oil or almond oil

1 teaspoon dried rosemary leaf (optional)

1 tablespoon dried yarrow flowers (optional)

¼ cup beeswax pastilles

Instructions

Soak the herbs in the olive oil; either combine the herb and the olive oil in a tightly closed jar and leave it 3-4 weeks shaking daily or heat the olive oil and the herb over very low heat in a double boiler for 3 hours until the oil is green. Pour through a cheese cloth to strain the herbs out and squeeze completely then throw the herbs. Heat the squeezed oil and beeswax in a double boiler until melted and mixed. Pour into lip chap tubes, small tins, glass jars and use on the rash. You can use it for stings, cuts, wounds or diaper rash.

Homemade Eczema Cream

Ingredients

½ cup shea butter

20 drops geranium essential oil

30 drops cedar wood essential oil

20 drops lavender essential oil

Instructions

Mix all the ingredients in a small jar and apply on the affected areas each night before bed.

DIY Homemade Eczema Cream

Ingredients

¼ cup coconut oil

¼ cup shea butter

15 drops lavender essential oil

5 drops tea tree essential oil

Instructions

Put water halfway full in a saucepan and heat over medium high heat but do not boil. Add the shea butter and the coconut oil in a Mason jar then place in the saucepan. Remove the Mason jar and allow it to cool slightly on the counter then add the essential oils. It's okay if the oil is warm when you add the essential oils, but it should not be hot. Mix your essential oil into shea/coconut mixture and then place the jar in the refrigerator until it gets firm. You can now use the eczema cream but if you would like more of a "whipped" body butter lotion, then put the oil in a kitchen stand mixer and mix on high for several minutes until the eczema cream looks like whipped butter. You may have to scrape the sides of the mixer down a few times. Apply liberally to any affected area of the skin.

This cream will liquefy if your house is warm, so you may decide to keep it in the fridge.

Other Essential Oil Recipes For The Skin

Soothe Dry Skin

Ingredients

12 drops myrrh essential oil

1 ounce virgin coconut oil (melted)

Instructions

Make a lotion using a 2% dilution of the myrrh essential oil in the virgin coconut oil. Use the lotion as required for moisturizing your skin.

Recipe To Balance Oily Skin

Ingredients

1 ounce aloe Vera

1 ounce witch hazel lotion

2 drops ylang ylang essential oil

6 drops juniper berry essential oil

12 lemongrass essential oil

Instructions

Mix all ingredients and store in a glass jar. Use daily as part of your skin care routine.

Sunburn Oil

Ingredients

20 drops lavender essential oil

4 ounces aloe Vera gel

Instructions

Combine the ingredients and apply the mixture on sunburned skin as often until it heals.

Stretch Mark Recipe

Ingredients

1 ounce virgin coconut oil

4 drops helichrysum essential oil

4 drops geranium essential oil

4 drops frankincense essential oil

4 drops lavender essential oil

Instructions

Combine all the essential oils with coconut oil. Apply this blend to your stretch marks daily. It takes a while to see the results so be patient.

Aging Spots Remedy

This cream will promote healing and rejuvenation and eliminate darker complexion

Ingredients

10 drops lavender essential oil

2% dilution ounce virgin coconut oil

10 drops frankincense essential oil

10 drops myrrh essential oil

Instructions

Combine the essential oils into the 2% virgin coconut oil and store in a glass jar. Apply on the affected areas.

Itchy Skin Remedy

Ingredients

1 ounce almond oil

3 drops peppermint essential oil

3 drops lavender essential oil

Instructions

Mix ingredients and gently apply the mixture on affected areas. This will relieve the itching and prevent breakouts.

Fungal Infection Cream

Ingredients

1 drop oregano essential oil

2 teaspoons Fractionated coconut oil

1 drop tea tree essential oil

1 drop lavender essential oil

Instructions

Add the essential oils to the coconut oil and mix well. Apply twice daily to the affected areas until it heals.

Essential Oil Recipes To Treat Your Body

We will look at different health problems and sicknesses that you can treat simply by use of essential oils.

Essential Oil Recipe For Constipation

To deal with constipation, a massage using this essential oil blend can be performed. Below is a treatment for the problem.

Ingredients

5 drops peppermint oil

10 drops lemon oil

15 drops Rosemary oil

30 ml jojoba oil

Instructions

Mix the ingredients in a glass jar. You should apply the oil over the lower abdomen in a clockwise manner. This can be done three times a day. If the symptoms still persist, contact your doctor.

Essential Oil Recipe For Treating Fever

Fever is a mechanism that your body embraces that helps fight off infections. If you allow it to get too high, it can cause problems such as delirium and seizures, which can in turn affect the brain. Below is an essential oil blend to deal with fever.

Ingredients

2 drops eucalyptus oil

1 drop Rosemary oil

15 ml evening primrose oil

2 drops peppermint oil

1 drop black pepper oil

1 drop tea tree oil

2 drops lavender oil

Instructions

Mix all of the ingredients above then massage the resulting oil to the soles of your feet, top of hands, and the temples.

Essential Oil Recipe For Treating Varicose Veins

Various veins appear as purple swollen veins that are visible through the skin. They are formed due to accumulation of blood in veins due to interruptions as it flows causing them to twist and swell. This can be very painful and uncomfortable. Use the following essential oil recipe to reduce the pain.

Ingredients

20 ml Almond oil

4 drops cypress essential oil

2 drops of wheat germ oil

4 drops of lavender oil

Instructions

Combine all these ingredients together. Massage the resulting essential oil from your feet upwards to your legs and then work your way up to the heart.

Essential Oil Recipe For Treating Sinusitis

This is an inflammation or infection caused by bacteria. It occurs in some of the sinus openings in the bones around the nose and eyes. This can be caused by poor mouth hygiene, allergies, cold, tonsils or flu. Some of the symptoms include nosebleed, coughs, nasal congestion, fatigue, headache, mild fever, pain around the eyes and sometimes ear pain. The following is a relief formula for sinusitis.

Ingredients

2 drops peppermint oil

2 drops Rosemary oil

1 drop Eucalyptus oil

1 drop thyme oil

Instructions

Add all these ingredients to boiling water and inhale the steam. After that, proceed on to make massage oil using the following:

2 drops of eucalyptus oil

1 drop of tea tree oil

3 drops of geranium oil

3 drops of Rosemary oil

2 drops of peppermint oil

Instructions

Mix all of these oils and add 10 ml of your preferred carrier oil such as olive oil, jojoba oil, sunflower oil, pumpkin seed oil or walnut oil and massage the resulting essential oil gently on the forehead, neck, on and around your nose, cheek bones and behind and in front of your ears.

Essential Oil Recipes For Sore Throat

Pharyngitis (sore throat) is an indicator of inflammation of your pharynx, which is the part between the back of your mouth and esophagus. The inflammation is mostly caused by a bacterial or viral infection. Below is a recipe you can use to treat it:

Ingredients

1 drop of tea tree essential oil

1 drop of lemon oil

4 drops of chamomile oil

1 drop of thyme essential oil

Instructions

Mix the above ingredients and dilute the resulting solution in 5 ml of a suitable essential oil. Massage the resulting essential oil on your neck and the part toward the back of your ears.

Steam Based Remedy For Inhalation

Ingredients

2 drops of eucalyptus

2 drops of lavender

1 drop of thyme oil

Instructions

Mix the ingredients in hot water. Cover your head with towel over a bowl with the mixture and inhale the steam. Keep your eyes closed as the steam might be irritating.

Essential Oil Recipe For Intestinal Ailments

Ingredients

2 drops peppermint oil

1 drop rosemary oil

1 drop clove oil

5ml vegetable carrier (choose)

1 drop chamomile

Instructions

Blend with 5ml of the vegetable carrier oil of your choice. Rub the resulting essential oil over the area of discomfort.

Essential Oil Recipe For Mouth Ulcers

Aphthous (mouth ulcers) come in form of tiny open sores that form on the tongue, in the mouth, the roof of the mouth, grooves between cheeks and gums and on the mucus membranes inside cheeks and lips. They are often caused by mild infections or even by a state of emotional stress or anxiety.

You can use a cotton bud dipped in tree oil essential oil for immediate ulcer relief. Apply it directly to the ulcer.

You can also create a mouthwash using essential oils for the ulcers. Below is a recipe for this method:

Ingredients

2 drops of tea tree oil

2 drops of thyme oil

2 drops of lemon oil

2 drops of geranium oil

2 drops of peppermint oil

1 glass of warm water

10 ml of brandy

Instructions

Mix the above ingredients and swish the mixture around in your mouth then spit it out. Repeat this with the remainder of the mixture, if any. You can create another mouthwash by combining 2 drops of tea tree essential oil with 5 ml of salt and mix them in 500 ml of warm boiled water.

Essential Oil Recipes To Treat Your Mind

Essential Oil Blends For Stress Relief

Stress is a reaction to a stimulus that often upsets your mental balance. If you have been experiencing stress, then you can try the following recipe for stress relief. You can choose one of the following blends below:

Blend 1

1 drop of Ylang Ylang oil

3 drops of grapefruit oil

1 drop of jasmine oil

Blend 2

3 drops of Clary sage oil

1 drop of lavender oil

1 drop of lemon oil

Blend 3

1 drop of Vetiver oil

2 drops of Roman chamomile oil

2 drops of lavender oil

Blend 4

1 drop of geranium essential oil

3 drops of bergamot oil

1 drop frankincense oil

Instructions

After making a selection of your choice of one of the above blends, proceed to choose a method below to use with the blend.

Massage Oil

-Multiply the blend you chose by two to total up to 10 drops.

-Mix with 1 fluid Ounce of carrier oil such as sunflower seed oil thoroughly

-Rub the resulting blend onto your body.

Diffuser Blend

Multiply the blend you picked by four to add up to a total of 20 drops. Mix the oils in a dark / tinted glass bottle. Ensure the oils mixes thoroughly by rolling the bottle between both of your hands. Take the required drops from the resulting blend to your diffuser. The number of drops are specified by the manufacturer of the diffuser.

Air Freshener

Multiply the blend of choice by six so as add up to 30 drops. Mix the drops with 3 Ounces of hydrosol/distilled water in a clean/new spray bottle. You can also choose to use 1.5 fluid Ounces of water/hydrosol with 1.5 ounces of high proof alcohol to make the aroma produced linger for longer. Do not fill the bottle to the top. This is done so as to allow space for effective shaking before use. You can spray it to your house for a sweet aroma that will leave you stress free.

Essential Oil Blends For Addressing Anger

Anger is an emotion emanating from the brain that is characterized by aggression towards something or someone. If not managed properly, it can lead to serious damage to the brain causing unexpected behaviors. You can calm your anger with a more natural way with use of essential oil blends. Below is a recipe that you can use to suppress your anger. Choose one of the blends below.

Blend 1

1 drop of jasmine oil

3 drops bergamot oil

1 drop Ylang Ylang oil

Blend 2

2 drops bergamot oil

1 drop Roman chamomile oil

2 drops of orange essential oil

Blend 3

3 drops of orange essential oil

1 drop rose oil

1 drop Vetiver essential oil

Blend 4

2 drops patchouli oil

3 drops orange essential oil

Instructions

Select any of the above recipes and mix all the ingredients in a dark glass bottle. Ensure you shake well. Proceed to follow any of the methods below for use.

Bath Oil

Add approximately 15 drops of the chosen blend to your normal bath oil. Mix it well and proceed to bath as usual.

Massage Oil

Mix 8 drops of the chosen blend with 20 ml of any carrier oil. You can use the resulting oil for a body massage.

Essential Oil Blends For Anxiety

Anxiety is a state of mental obsession, uneasiness, nervousness and apprehension or the concern about an event that is uncertain and can lead to panic attacks. This is often unpleasant to experience. If you often experience anxiety, then the recipe below is appropriate for you. You can use this recipe as a roll on oil or balm stick base.

Ensure that your skin is not sensitive to any of the following ingredients before you start.

Balm stick base

Ingredients

2 drops of sweet orange essential oil

0.15 ounces balm base

2 drops of geranium essential oil

1 drop of vetiver essential oil

Instructions

Mix all of the ingredients and put the resulting mixture in a tube. Apply to your temple and wrist pulse point as desired. Keep the remainder in your purse or pocket to use anywhere.

Roll-on oil

Ingredients

2 drops of neroli essential oil

0.33 ounces jojoba essential oil

3 drops bergamot essential

Instructions

Mix the ingredients in a roller bottle and apply on temple and wrist pulse points as required.

Do not apply this mixture just before you go out in sunlight or with sun tan units because the mixture is phototoxic.

Essential Oil Recipes For Treating Different Hair Problems

Essential Oil Recipe For Hair Loss And Baldness

There are a variety of ingredients that can help you fight hair loss, below are some;

Ingredients

4 drops of rosemary

4 drops Roman chamomile

6 drops of Clary sage

10 drops of lavender oil

40 drops of carrot seed oil

11 tablespoons of sweet almond

1 tablespoon jojoba

Instructions

Mix the above ingredients in a clean bottle by shaking well. Warm before you use. Apply the mixture into your scalp and leave it overnight. Repeat this for several weeks until you begin to see changes.

Essential Oil Recipe For Hair Growth

Ingredients

3 drops of geranium oil

6 drops of jojoba oil

100 ml mix of rosewater and distilled water on a 1:1 ratio

5 drops of rosemary oil

15 ml apple cider vinegar

3 drops of carrot oil

Instructions

Mix the ingredients well then massage about two teaspoons of the mixture into your scalp. This can be done in the morning just after washing and partly drying your hair. Ensure you massage with care so as to avoid stretching or breaking your hair. Keep the remainder in the fridge.

Essential Oil Recipe For Baldness

The following recipe can be used to fight baldness and restore hair growth.

Ingredients

2 drops of juniper oil

4 drops lavender oil

4 drops cypress oil

3 drops rosemary oil

1 drop frankincense oil

4 drops of cypress oil

2 drops of cinnamon essential oil

4 drops of geranium oil

Instructions

Mix all the ingredients thoroughly. Take only 1 drop of the mixture of essential oils each day and massage it to your scalp before you sleep. It is recommended that you dispense a single drop onto your finger. Rub the drop on all your fingers to distribute the oil. Later massage the scalp with your fingertips, concentrating mostly on the bald spots. You must repeat this treatment daily without skipping a single day.

If any irritations occur in your skin, cease the treatment immediately since you will be using undiluted pure essential oils that might cause sensitivity.

After completing the treatment, wash your hands thoroughly to avoid contact of the undiluted essential oil with your nose, eyes and other sensitive areas which might cause irritation.

Essential Oil Recipe For Alopecia

The following is a recipe to curb alopecia that can be mixed with your shampoo. You should not use more essential oil other than specified to avoid severe irritations.

Ingredients

2 drops of tea tree oil

8 drops carrot oil

7 drops of lavender oil

15 drops of jojoba oil

7 drops of rosemary oil

100 ml of the shampoo of choice preferably a mild one

Instructions

Mix the ingredients well. Wash your hair with the resulting mixture to curb alopecia. If you detect that your skin is irritated by this mixture you should stop the treatment.

Essential Oil Recipe For Tangled Hair

The following recipe conditions and detangles hair without leaving any residues. It can also control freezing for some types of hair.

Ingredients

20 drops of carrot seed oil (cold pressed)

20 drops of lavender

5 ml solubaliser or emulsifier

20 drops of rosemary

150 ml distilled water

Instructions

Put the distilled water in a spray bottle and add an emulsifier then shake well. Add the oils and then shake thoroughly again.

Spray just enough to dampen your hair (if dry). Gently comb or brush hair.

Oily Hair

Ingredients

2 tablespoons of grape seed

9 drops of Ylang Ylang

2 drops of rosemary

9 drops of lime

Mix all the above ingredients. Apply a tablespoon to your scalp and hair and massage it in. Give it time to penetrate overnight or for a few hours. Proceed to wash your hair with a natural unscented shampoo twice. Repeat this for three times a week.

Essential Oil Recipe For Dry Hair

Below are some recipes that can help to moisturize dry hair.

Hot oil treatment

This recipe is sufficient for a person with mid length hair. For longer hair, you might increase the quantities a bit.

You can substitute jojoba oil with cheaper carrier oils such as almond and coconut essential oil since jojoba oil is quite expensive.

Ingredients

2 drops of ylang ylang oil

3 drops of Roman chamomile oil

6 drops of sandalwood oil

1 ounce jojoba oil

Instructions

Mix all of the ingredients in a cup/bowl. Heat the mixture in the microwave until it is hot. Massage the hot oil directly to your hair. After you have finished, put on a shower cap and leave it on for about 30 minutes. The longer you let it stay that way, the more conditioned your hair will be.

Finally, wash all the oil out of your hair. Start by applying shampoo before you wet the hair, then wash and dry it in your usual way.

Recipe 2

Ingredients

6 drops of rosemary oil

½ ounce of sweet almond oil

1 egg yolk

1 ounce of raw honey (use raw honey as it possesses therapeutic properties that cannot be found in regular processed honey that you often find on store shelves)

Instructions

Beat the honey, egg yolk and sweet almond oil together; add the rosemary essential oil as you continue beating.

Wet your hair partially and then later apply the mixture. Put on a shower cap and leave the applied mixture to sit for roughly 30 minutes.

Wash and then dry you your hair normally.

Recipe 3

Ingredients

½ ounces of aloe Vera

4 ounces of distilled water

Choice of hair care essential oils like chamomile, rosemary or lavender (dilute between 10 and 20%)

Instructions

Put all the ingredients in a spray bottle and mix them thoroughly. Apply the mixture every time before you dry it with a hair dryer.

Conclusion

Thank you again for purchasing this book!

I hope you have found ways of addressing various health problems using essential oils. The next step is to start using essential oil recipes for a healthier you.

Thank you and good luck!

Printed in Great Britain
by Amazon